How to Lose Fat Faster

(And for Good!)

Mike Spagnola

Copyright © 2015 Mike Spagnola

ISBN: 1508806349

ISBN-13: 9781508806349

WWW.EDGESTRENGTH.COM

DEDICATION

This book is dedicated to the Edge Fitness & Performance
Family and the Edge Team.

*Edge Fitness & Performance is the premier results-based group
personal training facility located in Cary, Illinois. For more
information on how you can obtain your zero obligation
consultation, visit us at www.edgestrength.com or call us at
773-577-1190 and get started today.*

CONTENTS

www.edgestrength.com

MIKE SPAGNOLA

ACKNOWLEDGMENTS

Special Thanks to Matt Gerebizza and Samantha Spagnola for taking the time and effort to interview and create a great dialogue about these topics. Without them, the book would be half the substance and not have nearly the same impact on the results of all our readers. Thank you guys.

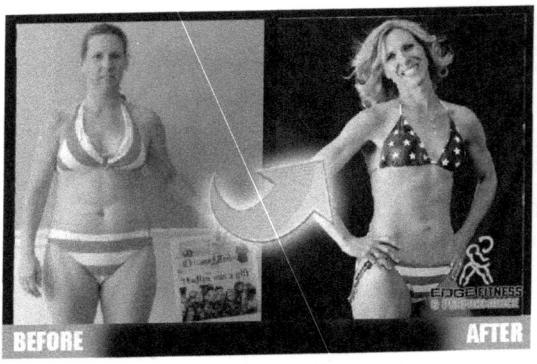

"I joined Edge Fitness and Performance just to get into a little better shape. From the beginning it was a good fit. Edge offers semi-private personal training sessions in a group setting. Owner/ Trainer Mike Spagnola, himself an accomplished strongman, has created group fitness training with individualized attention. Workouts are a perfect blend of resistance training and cardio with a focus on form and progress. Even though it is a group session, you get personal attention and workouts are targeted to individual fitness levels and you progress at your own pace. I was always challenged to perform at higher levels, and I began to see results in just 4 weeks. Mike combines his wealth of fitness/exercise knowledge with nutritional guidance to create the perfect formula for a total transformation of body, mind and life. At 49 years old, I am in the best shape of my life. I have lost 36 pounds, over 20 inches and 5 dress sizes in just 7 months. What do YOU have to lose?"

-Mary B.

1 FASTER FAT LOSS

How to Lose Fat Faster is a book that we built out of frustration from our clients at Edge Fitness and Performance and the struggles that they are having.

What constitutes good fat loss, at what rate they should be losing fat, how to lose fat, why fat loss should be a goal and... just taking things from there. Quite honestly, a big problem is people want to lose weight, when really their only goal and concern should be to lose fat. Losing weight is easy —you can lose muscle, bone, limbs, organs...but obviously that's not the goal, or the point.

When we talk about losing fat, we're talking about looking better—in clothes, in a swimwear, and naked. Let's be honest here...most people are training to be healthier, and to look better naked. Most people that say otherwise are just not telling the whole truth.

Exactly what constitutes fast fat loss:

Normal professionals would say anything from 1 to 2 pounds of weight is normal to aggressive fat loss and when it comes to losing fat it's really going to depend on the individual, but anywhere from 1 to 2 pounds a week of fat is going to be pretty fast fat loss. More beginner type individuals that are new to this type of training and eating are going to be able to lose upwards of that. The real kicker is that it's not about the weight...it's about the FAT loss. If you're losing fat, it's possible your weight doesn't budge much, and that's honestly okay. I don't know anyone who would complain about dropping 1-2 pant sizes in 6 weeks, regardless of their weight.

A big portion of this concept is to just forget abut the number itself. That number tells a (very incomplete) part of the story. How many people do you know that weigh 150lbs? How different do they look?

That's because height, muscle mass, bone density, bone structure, and body fat distribution all play a big role in how you look at a certain weight. What looks good one one person might look fabulous on another, and might look not-so-good on a third.

Fat Loss instead of Weight Loss is Key

Anyone can lose weight—as Dan John, a highly prominent strength coach, always says, "if you want to lose weight and cut off your left arm you will be down about 10 pounds". The idea is that we're not trying to lose weight; we're trying to lose fat. Fat is the stuff that make us not look as good, fats are the stuff that sit around the mid section, the thighs, love handles, etc.

So, when we are losing fat we are just revealing lean body mass or maintaining our bone density for health or maintaining our muscles for aesthetics and for function and then we're just getting rid of the fluff that we don't actually need to have on our bodies anymore.

This key difference is one of the reasons people who follow the concepts in this book experience such dramatic success when compared to some other methods. Other methods are OK with just weight loss. My question is this—if you can lose 20lbs of fat instead of 35lbs of fat, muscle, and other tissue, then why wouldn't you? Sure, it takes an approach that's definitely different then most people are used to, but you didn't open this book to learn the same old stuff now, did you?

Three components to focus on to lose fat

The three things that we need to focus on are:

1. Obviously **diet** is going to be a big number one to kick things off - that's going to be the first subject we focus on and, not unrelated, that's going to be the one that most people fall short on, so we are definitely diving into that. Do a quick search for "weight loss diets" on any search engine and you'll see why we have so many issues with this. Low fat is good, low carb is good, protein makes you bulky, sugar will kill you, grains are making you fat....the list goes on and on. If we legitimately tried to follow the warnings we read online, there would be absolutely no foods left to eat. One of the things that our coaching staff does, is this: we don't just say "alright eat this or eat this," with generic meal plans – there are a lot of them out there and from our experience these are short term solutions to long

term problems ...so that leads us into the second thing that we focus on.

2. **Building strong habits for fat loss**. Both with nutrition and training consistency we are trying to change habits because if we can change our activities on a day to day basis then we are going to change the type of outlook we have on fat loss, nutrition, and training. Then, and only then, are you going to be more likely not only to be successful, but to be successful long term, which is what we really want our clients to see. When we go over our initial orientation, our staff always talks about the "Jewel rule". That is, the last thing we want is to help you get the results you want, then see you a few years later shopping at Jewel back where you started. We want long term success through knowledge and application.

3. The third thing is **the type of training you're doing**. A lot of people go to the

gym and their preferred method of training consists of walking on the treadmill for a few minutes, doing all the machines and then they are done; so we talk about some of the stuff that we do at our gym, but more specifically we talk about the method of training that we use.

It's Metabolic Resistance Training and we will discuss how that is going to help not only burn fat faster, it's going to keep people's metabolism revved and it's going to keep lifting and training fun. The last thing, the fun in training, that's really important because the second working out stops being fun and it starts being a chore, you become a time bomb just waiting to quit or give up and, again, that's not what we want. We are looking for long term sustainable fat loss.

Special Tips Tricks, etc Coming Soon!

Yeah, so we are going to sprinkle some throughout the book – the special tips and tricks that will help you lose some fat faster. If there's one recommendation I can make, or one thing I can say is that as you go through this book, make sure you are taking notes and taking away some key points. Every page is going to be filled with information, so you will learn something with every turn, and all that's good... but there is definitely going to be some key takeaways. I would tell you what they are, but they are going to be different for each of you reading this. So, literally use the reading of this book as a new beginning; a start to building new habits.

Let that start now; what I would plan on doing is having a notebook next to this book as you read it and as you are going through it, grab some key takeaways or something that kind of hits you in the face like "wow, I should definitely do that," or "I should definitely be thinking of that"; that's when you want to go write that down and that's one of the pieces of information you're going to use when you start building your new habits. This one thing alone will get you well on your way to faster fat loss.

2 Five Nutrition Hacks for Fat Loss

What are five nutritional hacks for fat loss? If you were to narrow it down to five tricks or hacks for fat loss what would they be?

Well, and I'm sure for certain people it's been beaten to death already, but the first hack thatI would give to people is to start drinking more water.

Hack #1 Drink More Water, but Have a Plan of Attack

Here's the difference though. That's usually where fitness experts would stop and say that's enough "oh just drink more water thats a good thing". But we are going to go into a little bit more detail today though.

For example, if you are 200 pounds now and you are looking for how much water to drink, take that and multiply it by .5 and then you have 100 ounces of water per day.

That's great and that's definitely going to start you off on the right path but the problem with this equation is most people go through the day drinking a cup here...a cup there, and then they just kind of guess. I suppose this is because not many people have a good eye for what a 12-ounce cup or a 16-ounce cup is. I know I don't, and I've been doing this for quite a while.

1) One of the tricks that I like to give our clients is this. Instead of just winging it and drinking some water here or there, I suggest grabbing one twenty four or thirty two ounce hard plastic or metal water bottle, and the only water that counts for your water intake that we just figured out is the water that comes from that bottle. So that's rule 1 with the water bottle.

2) The second rule is you don't fill the water bottle up until it's all the way empty.

Like I said before typically the hard plastic or glass water bottles are going to come in 24 or 32 ounces, so for most people that's going to be between three or four of those water bottles completely (completely full to completely empty) per day. Before you go out and grab one, know your needs and your lifestyle. Here are some things to consider:

- Are you 200lbs or 120lbs? That's going to depend on what type of water bottle you get. If we're using our 200lb example to get to 100ounces of water each day, getting the 32 ounce bottle is only going to be 3 waters a day. Seems way easier then the same guy grabbing a 20ounce bottle and filling it up five times.

• But, let's say our example is in traveling sales, is in a car all day and can't get water refilled back up easily. He might be better off grabbing a 48ounce water bottle and keeping it on his passenger seat all day.

• Do what works best with your schedule most of the time. Don't worry about the other 15 to 20% of the time, because that's not where the bulk of your results will happen.

• So, you want to really set that up right away. It's not difficult to drink more water, just make the choice and have a plan. It's all laid out right here.

Whoever you are, whatever you weigh, however your lifestyle, you can and should immediately start drinking more water.

Hack #2: Eat closer to Nature Most of the time

The next trick and the next hack that I recommend is to start eating less steps away from nature as often as possible. Another way we could put that is: the closer something is to nature, the more likely it is that it is going to be good for you. This is also the trick I actually give to any of our younger clients, like our 10 year old clients. Honestly, sometimes these kids have some crazy ideas about what's good for you, what's not good for you, and a lot of that is thanks to marketing from certain companies and brands and things of that nature. What I tell them is this: "don't worry about the brands, don't worry about *anything else* other than if it's one step from nature then you probably can eat it pretty frequently, if it's two steps then it *should* be eating sometimes. Finally, if it's three steps away from nature, it doesn't mean never to eat it but it means that it's probably not helping your goals and you should eat it only a little bit." Let's give a couple examples of all of them.

Foods that are one step from nature. You want to think of these as foods you can basically see either in the wild or on a farm so we are talking meat, nuts, fruits, potatoes, and vegetables. You look at any of these foods and, without any knowledge of diet, nutrition, or health, you can probably assume that these are going to be better food choices, even if you might not know why. These are foods that'll fill around 60-70% of your diet depending on the day.

The next step are level two or step two foods. These are going to be the things that are two steps from nature. So in this group I like to include foods like whole wheat bread, rice, and pasta you can literally go find the wheat, which is one step from nature, and then is processed and cooked, making all of those things. Other items from this group are more complex foods that use multiple foods from group one, cheese, milk and other dairy products,things of that nature. All of these examples are going to be two steps from nature and they shouldn't be eaten all the time but they're going to be okay for you. Milk can really be considered a one step or two step food— it just depends on how it treats your stomach. Some people get on pretty easily drinking milk and some people don't, so the best way to handle that is on a highly individual case. If you tolerate milk (no breakouts, not stomach issues, or gastrointestinal issues) then it can be had on the regular. These are foods you'd eat 30% of the time, on average.

The last step (and that's the farthest step away from nature) is what you are going to eat pretty infrequently, or step three foods. Again, I don't think complete avoidance is a good protocol when it comes to eating, but challenge the foods you eat and demand more from them. How did an Oreo become an Oreo?

The answer to that, of course, is through magical deliciousness.

In all honesty, there is a lot of 'stuff' that happened for that to become a food. Cookies take a bunch of ingredients and all of a sudden it's food. Those are the types of things that you want to eat pretty infrequently; that's not to say you avoid them altogether, but rather than those making up the bulk of your diet, (which I think for a lot of us, that's exactly what we do), begin the process toward smarter food selection and begin to move a little bit closer to nature.

This step altogether won't guarantee everything you eat is healthy and to your fat loss goals. However, it will get you closer, and it will get you eating like an adult, which is a giant step in the right direction for many of us. After this step, everything else gets easier.

Hack #3: Moderation is Critical to your Success, but it's not What you Think

The third trick that we like to give our clients from Edge is to follow everything in moderation. What this isn't is a role call to eat garbage in moderation, but with the onset of paleo diets and other fads, we've basically been a huge pendulum shift in how people eat.

Before, we had people who were petrified of fat, so they were part of a super low fat craze. Everybody was higher carb as a result. The USDA guidelines/food pyramid we all love so much was primarily used to show people that they should have 200-400 grams of carb per day. The result? A lot of people gained a lot fat, and got over weight. Naturally its more difficult to take accountability for our poor eating habits then it is to explain how overeating, poor overall food choices on a long term basis, and poor habits are the cause of obesity, so we stopped blaming fat and we decided we should eat fat in abundance.

So now, we have a whole generation of fitness enthusiasts that go paleo or follow `Palaeolithic' principles which ends up being an all natural, high fat diet, and blaming all those carbs for the last generation's weight problem. This isn't a bad way to eat, and it might even sound similar to our last nutrition hack, eating closer to nature.

When we begin to talk about losing fat and energy intake, it is very, very easy to over eat, to manipulate unhealthy recipes into becoming paleo, thus making them healthy. I see this all the time with 'Paleo Cake' or 'Paleo chocolate chip cookies'. These are still chocolate chip cookies and are not healthy because they are paleo.

Another pretty common trend is to change up a recipe to lower the carb count, all the while adding several hundred calories in fat. One big way we see this happen is with making almond or coconut flour pancakes. Rather then replace the flour with something a little closer to nature, like oats, those fearing the carbs will add in upward of 300 calories per serving of fat to avoid 120 calories of carbs. This is backward thinking and will not help anyone lose fat faster, or for good. When that happens no matter what, and it doesn't matter if the excess calories are coming from paleo foods, it doesn't matter if the calories are coming from fats, and it doesn't matter if they're coming from carbs—the end result is that you store the excess energy (calories = energy) as body fat. This is obviously the opposite of the goal.

Now, a more moderate approach where we do not fear fat, carbs, or protein, but rather understand them as a food and energy, is a better approach. Teaching anyone to fear food is fast track to failure. I think we've all been there, done that. So, if that means once in a while eating a few oreos, so be it. Better eat something you know doesn't fit your goals once in a while then to fear an entire type of food.

Hack #4: Protein in Moderation, too. It doesn't Make you Bulky, and it Doesn't Build muscle.

Most people need more protein to get into a moderate intake level. We talked about fat, we talked about carbs, and I think the majority of us understand more about these simply because of all the fad diets I mentioned earlier. However, most people need to decrease those in order to get to a moderate level, whereas almost everyone i've ever met and helped get results needs to increase their protein intake. What I suggest in order to give yourself a general guideline to follow every day, is take *your body weight and multiply it by '.6' and then also multiply it by '1'.* That's going to give you a range that helps you decide about how much protein you should eat every day.

For example, we will use our same 200 pound example from before. For him to figure out how much protein he should take in each day, he would take .6 x 200 and that would give him 120 grams of protein for the lower end. On the other side, he take 200 x 1 giving him 200 grams of protein on the upper end. That means that our example should be having roughly 120 – 200 grams of protein every day. This is much less then some muscle guys who try to take in much more, and then much more then the USDA guidelines, (having 50 grams) which is just not enough to build and repair tissue like we want it to.

The other thing to say about protein is that protein alone does not build tissue; it just spares tissue from being wasted in the body. What that means is that when you are dieting you are going to start to lose tissue. The goal of course is to lose fat tissue, but what happens is you end up losing muscle tissue as a result and on a lower protein diet the likelihood is you will lose more muscle than you will anything else. On a low protein diet, the best case scenario is that you lose the two equally. Maintaining the protein intake that we recommend will virtually guarantee that any kind of muscle loss is kept to a minimum while you are dieting and losing fat.

Why is that important?

Simply put, if you don't have a little muscle, losing fat will just make you look skinny.   For some people, that may be enough, but most of us aren't looking to get thin; we want to be lean, fit, and look good, so we have to maintain just a little muscle to accomplish that.

The final trick and one that we have (kind of) alluded to the entire time is to follow the 80/20 rule. What that means in this case is that most of your results are going to come from 80% of what you are doing all the time. That means that if you eat twenty-eight meals per week (4 meals per day for the less math inclined), 80% of those meals should be on point. The rest of them can be a little bit `less then on point.' It doesn't mean that you can go and have a free-for-all and have five big, cheap meals, but if three to five of those meals each week don't fit into your diet perfectly or you have some foods that maybe don't fit into the tips and tricks that we just recommended, it's definitely not a deal breaker. If the other twenty-three meals are on point each week, then you are doing the things you need to do in order to lose fat.

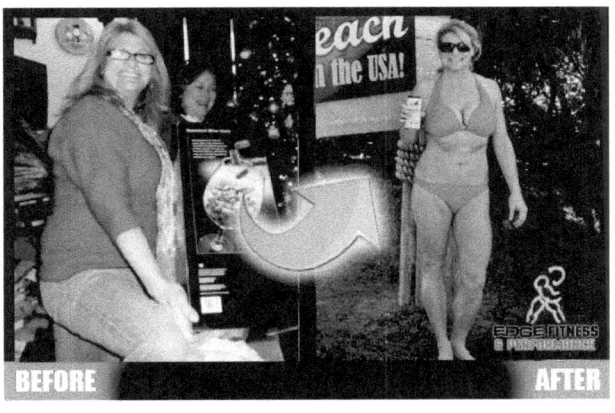

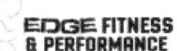

3 Metabolic Resistance Training

Metabolic Resistance Training (MRT) and how it will help you Lose Fat Faster.

Metabolic Resistance Training (MRT) is the concept that, rather than splitting our training into strength portion, and a muscle building portion, and a cardio portion, it is doing it all together at once. So, what we are doing is using weights, whether it is body weight, kettlebells, barbells, slides or ropes - whatever the implement is - but we are using weights to perform a cardio-based workout, and the end result is you burn more calories (and don't forget, fat is energy and energy is calories). You burn more calories during the actual workout, you burn more calories after the workout, and you also built just a little bit of lean muscle.

That way, as you are stripping the fat away (which is our overall goal here, right?) you are going to not only have a better body, you will have a speedier metabolism. Another bonus is that you are going to save time rather than splitting up your workouts into a bunch of different components.

The Best Type of Training for Fat Loss

At our gym we use Metabolic Resistance Training (MRT) we just explained. The idea behind that is simple. People are busy, people don't have a lot of time and to be honest, people are not patient for their results. The `old school' or conventional way of doing things would have a strength portion of their lift and then they would have a cardio portion. Then there is what you see people doing now in the gym. These good intentioned people will do tons of repetitions on various machines, and then they would do some treadmill jogging or stationary biking. As you can see, MRT isn't being widely used yet. At least, not in most gyms.

Now, we have a system and a logical structure for combining the best of both worlds and getting more bang for our buck in less time. We are building lean muscle, a calorie burning process itself, and then we're developing that extra lean muscle which, once it's on our body, burns calories more calories all the time.

One quick side note*— Everyone says muscle weighs more than fat. It doesn't weigh more, but it's denser, so the end result of having some lean muscle is that you can weigh more and look like you are much smaller. You will appear to *weigh much less than you actually do, and you'll be a metabolic nightmare, burning several hundred more calories throughout the day because you worked hard. Metabolic training accomplishes all of this.*

[Second quick side note* —Now, for those of you guys reading this who have the goal of bulking up or looking bigger/more muscular, the dieting factor (the fact that we're eating less calories than we need to build) means that we're not going to get big, and we're not going to get jacked from this type of training. This is especially true in a caloric deficit. Metabolic Resistance Training can be used to put on mass and minimize fat gain, but is best utilized with a strength training program, the diet is different, and this program is outside the context of this book—just know it can be done, just differently]

To wrap this up, you're going to lose fat, and you're going to have just that little bit of muscle to make your body look great.

The worst thing that could happen is you lose fat only to reveal a body you're still not happy with. Metabolic Resistance Training virtually guarantees that as you lose fat, you are developing a body you will love!

How our clients train when losing fat.

We do a hybrid style of training. What this means is we definitely have our metabolic days utilizing MRT, and they're super important. Our coaching staff has realized that the missing component in the metabolic resistance training puzzle is the resistance portion. The solution is to have MRT workouts that have more of the emphasis on the developing strength.

Our strength days are divided into the beginning/primary portion, which still is pretty fast-paced/metabolic, but we have one main movement that we focus on getting better at. This main movement is followed by one to three easier movements, and the purpose of these secondary moves is to help us get prepared for that main movement.

Example of a Metabolic Strength day:

A barbell dead lift for three sets of six reps. In between every set, we'll have our clients do a long lunge-hip stretch to open up and stretch the hip flexors. This ensures that the deadlift can be easily executed with a flatter back. Then we'll add some bridging on the ground to wake up/ activate those glutes. The benefit is twofold because most of our clients are sitting all day, so we give them an opportunity to loosen up their hips to strengthen and activate the glutes. That way, when they get back to their next set of deadlifts, it's going to look better. Then there's the added benefit that they are moving a little bit faster, keeping things metaboic. Now, they are burning more calories, aren't standing around for too long, which means they're keeping things metabolic. The end result is a metabolic workout while still getting that emphasis on the strength component, and helping fix a balance/postural issue related to a sedentary lifestyle.

One thing that people miss out on when they only do Metabolic Resistance Training is they tend to miss the boat on seeing any need to get stronger. If done correctly, MRT will absolutely get you stronger. Another way to understand this is to put it in terms of an actual workout you might do:

Lets say the MRT workout for that day calls for ten kettlebell swings, followed by ten bodyweight rows, followed by ten lunges each leg and you're doing as many rounds as you can in ten minutes. Now, imagine two people the same height and weight doing the same workout. However, person A is using a seventy five-pound kettlebell and person B is using a fifty-pound kettlebell.

Who is going to get more out of that workout?

If you answered person A, then you are absolutely correct! That person's MRT workout is going to be much more effective then person B.

That's why we break it up and have a strength-based day (which is still Metabolic Resistance Training with a heavy strength emphasis) and Metabolic Resistance Training day (which is very heavy on the metabolic side like I mentioned before). If we can get people safely moving more of their bodyweight, or heavier weights, or moving the weights easier and faster, then we are going to get them to burn fat faster as well.

The Profound Effect of Metabolic Resistance Training on Fat Loss

We alluded to it a little bit before, but it's definitely worth explaining in more detail. As you are doing a Metabolic Resistance Training session, you are burning calories, and typically you are buying more calories per minute then most other forms of exercise. But, the good stuff doesn't end there. You are also using your muscle mass in a way that signals our bodies to hold onto it. Simply put our bodies don't do what we want them to do, they do what we tell them to do and what we show them to do. If you're dieting to lose fat, then you need to give your body a reason to hang onto your muscle mass, and MRT accomplishes just that. So I guess in a way, muscle does have a `use it or lose it' kind of property, and this is especially true if you are not using your muscles and you are eating at a deficit (which means you are eating less calories than you need to sustain your body weight – which is what you need to lose fat).

Here's what ends up happening. Say that as you lose a pound of fat along with a half a pound of muscle or other lean tissue, so every three pounds you lose is two pounds of fat and one pound of muscle/ lean tissue. Now, what'll happen is that you'll get down to a certain weight thinking you will look a certain way, but you end up not looking as good or as appealing as you thought. This is because you've lost so much muscle on the way that now you need to get even smaller.

Metabolic Resistance Training changes that dramatically. This fat loss method is so effective, it doesn't just have a profound effect on fat loss, it has a profound effect on how much weight (because we're just burning fat) you need to lose in order to look your best and will actually give you the body you envisioned when you set out on your fat loss journey. So, it really does change the game on both levels.

Other Types of Training Methods that should be used for fat loss.

I think the only other type beyond Metabolic Resistance Training and the Metabolic Resistance Training with the strength deficits that can sometimes be used, is if a client likes to do a certain type of activity. At our gym we don't do yoga, pilates, dancing, jogging or any kind of running force but it doesn't mean that we tell our clients not to. If people enjoy those things and they're making them an addition to their main program, then we have no problem with people adding in some sort of activity. We just don't want people to have the wrong idea and think that that is the optimal way to train or to burn fat. What we are trying to do is to get people to have fun and if having a balanced program with a little bit less in optimal work is fun for them, pilates for another person or it might be a long distance jog, we're okay with that. As long as people are realizing that the Metabolic Resistance Training is where we are going to have the most profound effect on your body.

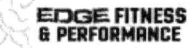

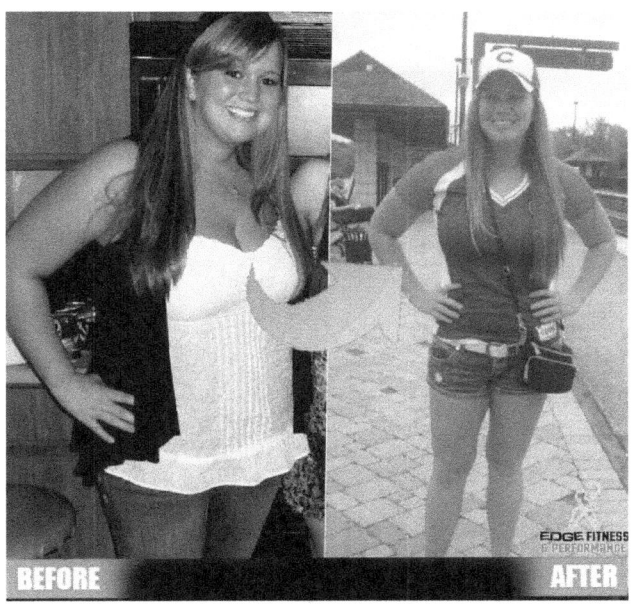

"[When I started…] I weighed in at 194 lbs. Breaking 200 was something I did not want to do! I've always lived an active lifestyle, playing a variety of sports since I was a kid, so working out wasn't the problem, but diet and correct working out was! Just like most of girls, I thought lifting heavy w/ low reps would make me bulky …little did I know it was the exact opposite! Four months after starting, I now weigh 176 lbs and hardly any clothes still fit me."

-Emilie K.

4 Proper Mindset for Massive Results

The Preferred Mindset for Fat Loss

For our clients, we focus on them having a growth based mindset. What that means is that they are focusing on progress every day, on celebrating little victories and for having long term success. It's really cool when you see "in six weeks I lost 35 pounds..or lose 10lbs in a week" but you always have to question what is going to happen in the next six weeks. Usually the answer to that question is that they unfortunately the one who lost 35lbs will end up gaining 40lbs, and the one who lost 10lbs will put that right back on as well. It's really hard to have that long term hundred percent grind. To be honest, one hundred percent effort and energy expended all the time, is a failure sort of mentality and focus when it comes to burning fat (and, I would suggest any venture worth enduring, although most of them are outside the context of this book). It's really a lifestyle enhancement, so we focus on going into any new fat loss journey with that mindset.

Where I believe people miss the boat when it comes to what a lifestyle means is they don't apply the growth mindset. They think, "oh it's my new lifestyle, I can't have that cookie", or " I don't want to go out and have a drink or two because my new lifestyle is *healthy"*. First, constant deprivation isn't healthy, it makes you a time bomb waiting to fail. Second, and more important to our long term success, someone who understands the growth mindset will say "I can go out, but I don't want to", or "I'll go out and have 2 drinks, but they will be lower calorie and i'll eat my protein earlier in the day since there won't be any good foods at the bar". That is the example of success; of having your cake and eating it, too.

For additional reading on the growth mindset, and how it applies to your entire life, there is a book out titled, of course, "The Growth Mindset" that some people would do well to read. If not, just remember that you're on a journey, not a quick adjustment that if you fail you've failed. At risk of sounding a little cliche, the only failure in fat loss is giving up.

How to Handle a Lack of Motivation When it Hits

I think that motivation is, in a way, overplayed. Before you get up in arms about that, because it definitely sounds blasphemous coming from a fitness professional, hear me out. What we really need to focus on is the idea that motivation is simply an emotion. It is something that is fleeting, it's just like being happy, sad, mad, or glad...the long story short is that motivation goes away not just eventually, but usually pretty quickly. I'll be honest when I say that motivation is super valuable for getting a new client started; it's something that we need to capitalize on because that feel good feeling we call motivation is certainly what'll get someone from the couch to the gym.

If you feel the motivation that you're ready to lose weight, you should absolutely take that by the reigns and you should start to lose weight...you should get on that journey—on any journey, really. The warning and thing I want you to recognize is eventually that fleeting emotion we call motivation, just like every emotion, eventually goes away. And the thing about motivation is that when it's gone, it's gone. That's not so much the problem, but the fact that most people do the seemingly logical thing and try to find it again. This is a mistake, and both our clients and pretty much everyone reading this would be better off served focusing on becoming driven towards a goal instead of find that that lovely motivated feeling.

When you have drive to accomplish something, you wake up and you get it done because it needs to be done. It becomes important to you, and you make the decision to work toward it. Sometimes it ends up being fun, sometimes it doesn't, but the goal is to get to the point and the mindset where you don't do it because you felt awesome about it—you do it because you'll feel awesome about the end goal; about losing the fat and revealing the body you've always wanted.

The idea that you will always feel awesome while working out and dieting is a myth. Nobody feels awesome about everything all the time. One thing that does feel awesome is being lean, losing fat, and accomplishing a lifetime goal. That feels better then any emotion or motivated feeling. There's a commercial out there that says "do what you love, and you will never work a day in your life". While good-intentioned, the reality is that, love it or not, sometimes it still feels like work. Now, there are ways around this, and at Edge Fitness & Performance, we do everything we can do make sure our clients are having fun the entire time and staying true to the process (from switching up workouts, to coaching challenging and new/fun moves, to checking in on them outside of the gym, to having outings and creating a true culture that people come to look forward to. Our goal is to be the best part of our client's day, every day). The difference is that, armed with a growth mindset, you will have the drive and the determination to get a certain thing done so you ignore the lack of motivation. That's exactly the mentality that we need our clients to have and that we need to have if we are going to lose weight.

Tips and tricks for people to train or work out with more consistency.

1. The first thing is to s**chedule it like it's important**. You wouldn't blow off a lunch date with your mom if you hadn't seen her in six months, because you would have it written down, you would have it on a calendar app in your phone, you would have a reminder set, and you would probably

be excited for it. Now, you can't always guarantee you're going to be excited about a workout, and if you are working out two to four times a week, then obviously it's not a monumental event each time. This means that the only other option is to write it down and to schedule it. What gets scheduled gets done, and what gets done and what gets tracked gets improved upon.

2. The second thing is to **track your actual workout**. Let's say you go in and you're working on pull ups and kettlebell swings that day. You leave the gym, and there are a thousand and one other pulls on your life, so you virtually forget what you did by the drive home. Next week, we get ready to do a similar workout that we are progressing from last week. Well, how much weight did you use? How good was your form? Did you feel like you

were using your glutes (read: butt muscles) while you did the kettlebell swings? How about the pull ups? Were you able to do a row variation? Did you get your first ever pull up (okay, so you might remember this, but you also might not if you have been doing pull ups for 6 weeks...how many did you do in your last workout?) These are the types of things to track and that will help you be more consistent because now, rather than just be like "oh this workout will help me burn calories to lose fat you are working towards something else while you are working towards losing fat. That's going to keep you consistent throughout your journey.

Here's a sample workout from one of my clients journals:

1/24/2015 — 146lbs

A1 Squat   3x8 with 105lbs

A2 Plank 3 x 30 seconds (used 10lbs of weight)

B1 RDL 4 x 10 95lbs (first time using this weight!)

B2 Grappler situp 4x 10 each side

Finisher: Sled sprint 6 x 50 feet with 1 plate on sled

This probably took her 30 seconds to write down, but now she knows what date she worked out on, what she weighed (she's down 15lbs in the last 7 weeks!), what moves she did, and how well she did. There were a few notes in there so she can refer back. Some of them may or may not be used next week, but either way, 30 seconds of extra work and now she has a record of this workout forever. Pretty good trade off for someone serious about losing fat and getting the body they want and deserve!

How my Clients Stick to their Diets

The ones who are most successful are the ones who track what they are eating. We have people who just eat healthy for the sake of eating healthy, and they usually end up getting pretty lean. However, I'll be honest and say that they never get as lean as they want to. I believe this is because they are not tracking and they are not focusing their efforts on the balance that we mentioned earlier. If these clients continued eating proper foods, but began tracking to focus on fat, protein and carbohydrates, they'd get much faster and better results. In order to get lean, you need to have a plan.

The plan that we usually give people is to take, like we recommended before.

Protein: To figure out how much protein you should be eating each day, simply take .6 and 1.0 and multiply that times your body weight. This will give you a range for the amount of grams of protein you should eat each day.

Protein sources I like: Chicken, lean beef, lean pork, canned tuna and chicken, fish, shrimp, cottage cheese, greek yogurt, protein powder, and egg whites.

Carbs: For carbohydrates, take .6 and 1.0 and multiply by your bodyweight as well. The difference between protein and carbs is that this isn't a range. Instead, this is going to give you how many carbs you eat on a workout day, and how many carbs you eat on a non-workout day. On an off day, you will eat .6 x your bodyweight in grams of carbs, and on your workout day you will eat 1.0 times your bodyweight.

One quick note on maximizing your carb intake on workout days. You want to eat those carbs around your workout. So, a two hour window before and a two hour window after you workout should be where most of those carbs are eaten.

Carbs I like: Rice (brown, white, jasmine), whole wheat pasta, sweet potatoes, red potatoes, white potatoes, fruit (limit 2 per day), and whole wheat bread (limit 2 per day).

Fat: To figure out how much fat you should be eating, take your bodyweight and multiply it by .3 and .5. Eat the higher amount of fat on your off/non-workout days and eat the lower amount on workout days.

Fats I like: Olive oil, avocados, egg yolk/ whole egg, coconut oil, butter sparingly...all other fat in your diet should come from your protein intake (example: eating lean beef still has 5 grams of fat per serving).

Let's take our 200 pound example and figure out what he should be doing.

Workout Day:

Fat: (.3 x 200) = 67 grams of fat

Carbs: (1.0 x 200) = 200 grams of carbs

Protein: (.6 x 200 and 1.0 x 200) = 120grams to 200grams of protein

Non Workout/'Off' Day:

Fat: (.5 x 200) = 100 grams of fat

Carbs: (.6 x 200) = 120 grams of carbs

Protein: (.6 x 200 and 1.0 x 200) = 120grams to 200grams of protein

If you're confused about having to track two different types of numbers on different days, I would recommend just going right in the middle and eating the same each day. The above example will yield better results, but if it's too complicated and you struggle tracking each day because of it, I would just keep it more simple.

Every Day Tracking (for simplicity)

Fat: (.4 x 200) = 80 grams of fat every day

Carbs: (.8 x 200) = 160grams of carbs every day

Protein: (.6 x 200 and 1.0 x 200) = 120grams to 200grams of protein every day

This isn't as specific as our first example, but will still yield much better results then guessing on your diet each day.

Tracking is what is going to help people have long term success and see the results are looking to achieve. One quick note on this: the people who are tracking, even if they are tracking an imperfect diet, are still going to get better results. This is because they are going to be able to build upon that imperfect diet. The worst thing that we have to handle is when we see someone who thinks they are doing really well on their diet, and it turns out they are not getting the results. Usually, these people are not drinking, eating pretty good quality food, but the amounts aren't right for fat loss. This is frustrating for everyone involved, it also makes it very difficult for anyone to get help and progress along, simply because we don't have an actual sample of what they are doing. In this case, we don't really know where to go to help them until they are willing to help themselves little bit.

If you have a coach willing to help you, or if you are interested in actually losing fat for good, you have to be tracking. We recommend phone applications like Calo*rie Counter by Fat Secret*, *My Fitness Pal*, or *Lose It*. All of those are good apps that will help you to track your food, which by now you should realize will have you burning fat faster.

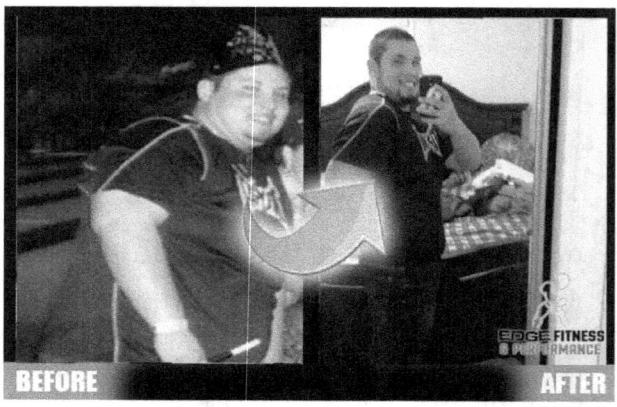

"Before Training at Edge, I was overweight, had very
little self-confidence, and didn't have the direction or
focus I needed. I tipped the scales at over 350lbs. When I
joined I knew two things: I weighed 350lbs and I
wouldn't stop working until I wasn't anywhere near
that. Best decision I've ever made, period. I have lost
over 120lbs, over 35 inches, 10 inches off my waist, and
have gained so much more. I passed the police POWER
test with flying colors, something I wouldn't have ever
been able to do a year ago, and something I need to do in
order to become a police officer for my career. I compete
in strongman competitions, can run 5+ miles, and am
much more confident that I can do whatever I set my
mind to."

-Rudy E.

5 Goal Setting for Fat Loss

Exactly what should my goal for fat loss be? How do you set a proper goal? What does that look like?

To set a proper goal you need to know exactly what you are hoping to accomplish. This might sound like an obvious statement, but its actually very common for a person to know they have to make a change, but not realize how much, how fast, etc. Its honestly no wonder why people have such a difficult time losing fat. The kicker is that this goal and pace could change throughout your fat loss journey, but when you set out you should have a very clear objective. Not only will it give you focus if you get off track, it'll help reshape your new goals because you'll be aware of your own growth in the gym and your diet habits in the kitchen.

We'll use one of our clients to explain how this process can be very powerful, and we'll call him Bill for this example. Bill came in at 325 pounds and he knew that he needed to weigh 240 pounds within a year, and additionally was going to pass a very physical test in order to get a new job that would be the start of his career. To me, that's a pretty powerful goal. It has all the components that you need for success. It has a very concrete number, it has a very important driving component - he's doing it not only to better himself and better his career but also for his family, for his kid and also for his wife. The one thing it didn't have (that we worked on) was to set a date on it (he said within a year, but we found out the first test was actually 11 months out, so we tracked and planned his goal for him to make it realistic, achievable, and measurable).

Now, I used that one last because setting a date on it sometimes is a recipe for disaster for some people. This is because if you set a date that's either insanely difficult to accomplish, or insanely liberal and far too simple of a goal, a few things will happen. If the goal is too unrealistic in that amount of time, you'll get discouraged because you fell short. An example of this is that someone sets out to lose 50 pounds in four months.

This is technically achievable, but it's extremely aggressive. Now lets say that person who set out to lose the 50lbs fall short by only losing 40 pounds. Quick show of hands on who would want to lose 40lbs in 4 months! While this person should be celebrating and recognizing what a massive success they just created for their life, they instead feel as if they fell short on their goal. What we like to do in this case, is scale a member's goal back just a little bit, because that will ensure not only success, but having that growth and positive and confident mindset. Our gym operates under the philosophy that doing this, while counterintuitive, will actually keep our clients losing weight and also maintaining it for years to come and ideally, for good.

Remember, fat loss is not just about losing fat, it is about losing fat and **then keeping it off.**

To re-cap, in order to have a proper goal for fat loss, you want to **have a date set. That date is one you want to be pretty aggressive, but not overly aggressive to the point of setting yourself up for failure.** You want to have **a strong reason why** (in Bill's case, it's the start to his career, which he'll use to better support his family—how much more powerful of a reason 'why' can you get?) and you want to have some **very clear parameters that you can measure success.** Again, in Bill's case, this was to lose 85lbs in 11 months and to pass a physical test, all of which are measurable and concise.

The last thing that we would look for is going to be mini goals set up along the journey. So, if your goal is to lose 100 pounds, you don't just set 100 pounds in eighteen months; you would say, "100 pounds in eighteen months is the overall goal, but at nine months I would like to have 55 pounds of fat lost; at six months I would like to have 35 pounds loss... six weeks from now I would like to be 10 pounds down" and so on. Whatever the parameters are, they should align with your overall goal and set you up for continued success. Setting up a bunch of mini goals that you can check and see if you are doing is critical for growing and getting closer toward obtaining the body you want and deserve. The nice thing is that if you fall short on those mini goals, you don't have to despair or feel like you failed—you simply know you've just got to prepare and work a little more for the next mini-goal check in.

Tracking Progress and When it's time to Switch it up

Progress isn't linear when it comes to fat loss. Put another way, there will be weeks when you step on the scale, feel like you did everything right and you only lost half a pound, and other weeks where you surprise yourself by losing an extra half a pound. Here's the thing that is super important to remember about fat loss though; half a pound a week over the course of a year still looks like 26 pounds lost. Twenty six pounds of pure fat loss on any person is going to look pretty awesome at the end of that year. Having the growth mindset, having concrete goals, and understanding that tracking and measuring progress to lose half a pound a week pays off huge a year from now.

Think about this time last year. Did you weigh the same? Did you weigh even less? How close does a year ago seem when you think about it backward? Like just yesterday! The problem is that when we look forward, we see what we have left to go through, and it seems difficult and daunting for "just" 26lbs lost. But rest assured when you look back to this moment right now, you'll wish you took this advice.

In order to track your progress and do a real 'self-audit' on your progress or lack thereof is to really ask yourself *"am I not progressing anymore?"* or *"am I just progressing slower than I'm used to?"* At a certain point you will start to progress slower, but don't fear that. This simply means that's when being consistent, following the rules that we set up earlier, and having that confidence in yourself and in the program are critical for long term success. if you were losing 2-4lbs the first 8 weeks, but then it slows down to .5 to a lb each week, don't fear or worry—be happy that you are following something so powerful and so consistently that you are closing in achieving the body you want and deserve!

The second thing is **if you consistently are not losing fat for three weeks, then it actually is time to change things up.** This means that if the scale is not moving, you are not getting leaner in your progress pictures, if your waistline is not smaller/inches and measurements are not moving forward, then it's time to move something around and make a change. Now, that could be an extra session, an extra walk per week, it could be an extra high intensity cardio or sprint workout. It could be twenty five minutes jog or it could be taking some calories out of your diet. The only way to tell is from working with a professional and like we've suggested, and, like this process all comes back to, tracking both your workouts and your nutrition throughout the days, weeks, and months.

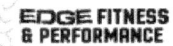

6 How Progress In the Gym Carries Over to Progress in Your Transformation

How We Define Gym Progress

One of the main ways that we define progress in our gym is by having clients progressively track their strength gains. Now, one of the things that people don't realize is about the process of losing fat is that getting stronger is a direct way to get leaner. Basically, when you look at how our bodies actually burn calories, especially with Metabolic Resistance Training like we went over in an earlier chapter, it's pretty simple to see how more weight in your hand throughout that entire process you will end up burning more calories.

The fact is, our program often fills the missing link in most people's fat loss journey. They come to us frustrated, doing things (mostly) the right way, and at a loss because they just can't lose fat…

…Then we take a look at their diet and realize they are rarely getting the right balance of fat, carbs, and protein, and that's step one to fixing their plateau. But the next step, and often the one that people haven't ever heard of in their entire lives (because, let's be honest and say that most of us know our diets are messed up, and need to be fixed to keep losing fat and to be healthy) is that they need to get stronger and challenge their muscles to grow and become fat burning machines.

I am amazed at the amount of clients that have come from bootcamp, personal training, or even group training backgrounds that still don't realize that a little bit of getting stronger and lean muscle goes a long way in their fat loss journey. It's fun because we get results and start drastically changing both our member's bodies, and also their mentality on what it takes to get in shape.

Progress will translate to increased fat loss.

The easiest way to describe this is to give an example. Let's say we have twin sisters fresh out of college. They ate the same for the last 4 years, did the same recreational sports, and so they are relatively the same body fat percent, muscle mass, weight, etc (the point of the example is that these people are beginning a workout with the same "starting point").

Now we'll have our twins do different workouts for 3-4 months. One will do MRT with a little emphasis on getting stronger, and the other will do cardio based stuff that burns a bunch of calories (although this statement is tricky because both the workouts burn a ton of calories, one just 'feels' harder). Then we have them do a fat blasting kettlebell swing workout. The one who worked on MRT and strength grabs a 50 pound kettlebell and swings it the whole time, while the one who did cardio stuff grabs a 30. Here's the not-so-trick-question: which is going to be more effective and which is going to burn more calories both during the workout and after?

If you guessed our stronger, 50 pound kettlebell swinging lady, you're right! Not only that, but the 50 pounds is working hard to sculpt her butt, her thighs, and her abs. It's pretty easy to see that the one swinging the 50 pound kettlebell is going to have a much more efficient, much more fat-burning workout than the person swinging the 30, and the only way to get to swing that 50 pound kettlebell is to progressively be getting stronger.

Another simpler way to explain this concept is that getting stronger and MRT opens up more options for you to burn more calories with every movement you do. You'll be able to do more with less effort, and burn more calories.

Lifting more weights burns more calories.

When you lift weights, you burn calories. When you utilize MRT, you lift weights and do other cardio type moves together. This revs up the metabolism like crazy. So now you're burning calories during the workout just like a cardio session (running, stair stepping, elliptical). And to top it off, you're also working on developing lean muscle so as you lose fat, you look even better Great, right?

But, it gets better. The process of breaking down muscles and getting stronger is taxing. All that means for us is that our bodies need even more calories to repair and refuel those muscles we just worked out. The result is that for the next 24-48 hours, you will burn even MORE calories then if you didn't do the workout. You basically turn your body into a "metabolic nightmare" and burn a more calories during the workout and after it. For most of us that workout 3-4x per week, this means that most of your week is spent in this higher fat burning phase.

Other ways to track progress in the gym.

Some of the ways that we'll also track progress is by getting faster at our workouts. You can't always move up in weight each workout, but we still want to get better someway, somehow. What we will sometimes have is workouts for time, which opens up a new option for us to measure our progress. We can then move the amount of repetitions we do in that given amount of time up each workout. If we have 40 seconds to get as many squats as possible, maybe we can't move up weight, but can we get another rep or two more then last week? If so, then you GOT BETTER. Congratulations!

One quick closing note:

Burning fat is great, but the habit of tracking your calories and tracking your workouts and your in-the-gym progress is honestly going to be more important and more valuable and bring more to the table on the long term. Once you learn how to do these, the habits can be cemented and you will not only lose fat, but you'll have a framework for long term success that will last a lifetime.

7 Drink your way to Fat Loss

Do you make your clients 21 and over refrain from alcohol completely?

One of the things we do at Edge is try to balance people's life with their fat loss goals. We have, and encourage our clients to create, realistic expectations of their own progress in terms of fat loss and contrast that with what they are realistically able to accomplish. For example, it is pretty unrealistic to ask someone who is a casual drinker two to three nights per week, or a "one or two" every night of the week to go from their current habits to drinking absolutely no alcohol. Rather than do that, we ask people to follow a couple of rules. These rules are critical for drinking on a diet and not gaining fat, and are actually pretty simple to follow:

Rule #1: Have no sweetened drinks. So, if you are adding any mixtures to hard liquor they should be diet or zero-type calorie drinks (think jack and diet, vodka and DIET tonic—that last one is important because most tonic water is actually sweetened. If you're cool with the bartender or if you're at a house, ask. If not, pick a different beverage to sip on). If you are having mixed drinks make sure that they are nothing like a long island or pina colada; both of those drinks, and pretty much any 'summer time sipping' drink are going to add a boat load of sugar and, more importantly, calories! Our bodies can handle the extra calories from alcohol if it's on occasion, but not from the extra sugar those drinks use to shuttle the booze into your mouth.

Rule #2: The other two options are beer and wine. People like to harp on them as being high in sugar or more fattening, but they're wrong. As long as you are not drinking them in excess, just like with any sort of zero calorie mixed drink, including excessively throughout the week and throughout the month, then it shouldn't really disrupt your fat loss.

Rule #3: Rule number three is to not eat while you're drinking. This one may be pretty tough depending on the gathering or event you're at, but usually we over eat poor choices while we are drinking alcohol. And then, of course, we blame the alcohol.

So, in short, no we do not make our clients refrain completely.

Let's settle this once and for all: Drinking and Fat Gain.

On its own – it's not gonna happen. It's actually pretty hard to drink enough calories to go over your daily calorie limit. For example, let's go back to our 200 pound male example who can probably eat roughly 2500 to 3000 calories a day without gaining weight. It would be pretty tough for him to drink 1500 calories on the drinks we recommend. This is especially true if he knew he was going out that night to have a few drinks, and controlled his eating earlier in the day. The one thing that is guaranteed to make any trainee gain weight is breaking rule number three, and eating while you drink. Whether you are at home drinking wine, out with buddies drinking some beers, or at a social event or party drinking some mixed drinks, there is going to be some food that goes along with that event. While the alcohol alone isn't going to make you fat, it definitely lowers our inhibitions when it comes to (well, all things but especially) food. It makes bad food more enjoyable by taking out all the guilt/realization that you're not losing fat. The end result? You just added an extra week or two of strict eating to accomplish your goals.

One quick note on drinking alcohol, even the way we recommend:

When you are drinking, you are not going to be burning fat. What you should expect for the entire night and maybe the entire next day is to put your fat loss on hold. However, if you can confine it to following our basic drinking rules, just drinking alcohol, (and again, that's hard liquor mixed with diet or zero mixer, beer, or wine) then you should still be able to reach all your fat loss goals or giving up something that you enjoy completely.

Managing Fat Loss and Still Enjoying a few Drinks.

First we set up a few parameters. The one thing is: on the day you are going to be drinking, recognize that you are not going to be losing fat and you are now in maintenance mode for a short period of time. Your new goal is to simply stop yourself from gaining any fat; you are going to stop any backwards progress. The first thing you are going to do is lower your intake for the rest of that day. If you know you are going out on a Friday night, then your first two or three meals for that day are going to be mostly protein-based with added vegetables to fill you up. This means you are now going low calorie that day while still providing your protein intake and a feeling of fullness. That way, as you transcend into what we'll call our 'drinking phase' of the night, you are not having a bunch of extra calories already. That clears up a little bit of calories for you to play around with and not burn fat, but at least not be gaining fat on that day.

For our clients at Edge, one of the things that we tell them is that they probably can't keep their old drinking habits, but they can definitely rebuild some new ones and still enjoy a social occasion, on occasion. Some common tweaks we make with our clients include:

1.   Switching from a one to two drinks a night to one drink 4-5x/week.

2. Mixing sugary drinks to dropping the extra sugar (you're going to drink alcohol but worry about the chemicals in a diet soda?)

3. Switch a 2x/weekend partier to a 1x/weekend partier (where we define

partier as getting drink (3). Drank (5). Drunk (6+ each night).

4. Making our clients realize that a "drink a night" or "a few drinks once a month" still makes you a "drinker". It's not a bad thing, but if you don't recognize your own alcohol consumption, you can't regulate, moderate, or control it.

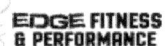

"In the first picture, I thought I was "in shape." I did what everyone taught me to do to lose weight...run. I ate as little as possible and was running miles a day. Then I met Mike and all the "founders" of Edge. My whole concept of fitness changed by working and talking with him. Working with the Edge Team has been a life changer for me. From the before and after pictures, I have dropped over 40lbs (From 290 to 248) and put on much more muscle... Without having met the amazing people at Edge, I don't think I would have ever had the courage to move away from my family and pursue my career and travel the world (even though he didn't agree with it, but friends never want you to leave).

Without everyone at Edge, I honestly couldn't say I would be the person I am today, both mind and body.

-Shane C.

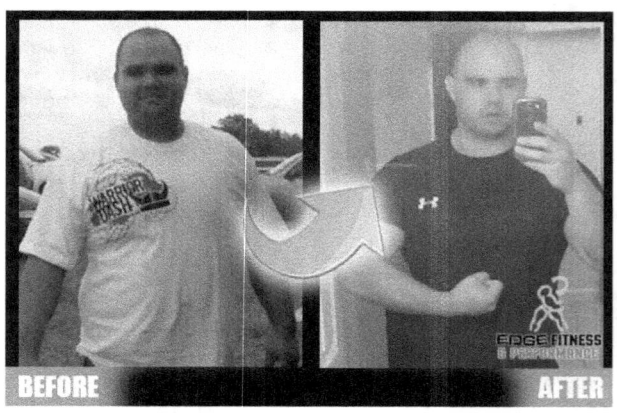

8 Why Regular Cardio Isn't Optimal for Fat Loss

What type of movements we Consider Regular Cardio.

Another term for what we are calling regular cardio is actually a term known as steady state cardio. Regardless of what we call it, cardio is anything we are doing for a low to middle intensity for 20-60 minutes or more. Low or medium intensity is moving at a pace with elevated breathing while being able to hold a normal or somewhat labored conversation. There are definitely more scientific ways of approaching this, but all you need to know is if you can hold a conversation, even a difficult one, you are very likely doing this type of 'steady state' cardio.

As far as the methods for doing this type of 'regular' cardio, it to be anything that you would normally see in a normal gym. Usually when you walk into the bigger health clubs, there are rows and rows machines designed for this from stair steppers, treadmills, ellipticals, and recumbent bikes.

Why isn't cardio good for fat loss?

To be honest, it's not that cardio is bad for fat loss. I mean, if someone is choosing between not moving and doing steady state type cardio, by all means they should hop on a treadmill and walk or run for their lives! It's just that there is a better way. If you recall from the past chapters, two main components of fat loss are:

1) preserving lean muscle mass through the proper training and nutrition.

2) burning calories/taking in less calories then you burn.

Now, in traditional philosophies, you will use cardio strictly for the fat loss. The difference between this and MRT is you have to put in just as much work and just as much time in simply maintaining your muscle mass with traditional weight training types of training. So now you have a 30 – 60 minute strength or muscle building session, and *then* you have a 25 – 60 minute cardio or fat loss session. With *Metabolic Resistance Training* we combine the best of both worlds and do both cardio and strength or muscle building/

maintaining at once. So it's not that cardio is bad for fat loss, it's just inefficient compared to MRT. Look, i'm the workout guy and I still want efficiency to get in and get back out.

One other key point that I should mention is that in order to have the same benefits that *Metabolic Resistance Training* gives anyone that is training, that regular cardio does not give you, is the additional calories that are burned after you are done with your sessions. If you are spending an hour lifting weight and then another 20-45 minutes doing cardio, this will be accomplished. However, when using solely traditional cardio and not weight training at all, the calorie burning process works like this: you start the activity, you burn calories throughout the activity, and then when you are done, you pretty much stop burning calories. When you choose to use your muscle mass to perform cardio-type movements like we do when we do a

Metabolic Resistance Training session, not only are you going to burn more calories throughout the duration of the workout (and very likely a higher amount of calorie per minute worked vs a treadmill or stair climber) but you are also going to burn calories for 12 to 36 hours after the workout is over, which ends up giving you much more bang for your buck. Again, more fat burned...more calories burned...in less time.

It all comes down to priorities, honestly. Like most of you, my time is limited (no, I don't spend all day working out just because I own a gym!) and if my primary goal is to be burning fat, i'm going for MRT most of the time. If you enjoy being in the gym and that is your life, then you probably shouldn't do much MRT, because it'll be far too efficient and you won't be able to spend as much time working out.

Regular Cardio: Good or Bad?

No, I think that if people enjoy doing it, whether it's a dancing class or a 30-minute jog or blasting away on the elliptical, they should by all means they do it; however, it's definitely not a) a necessity or b) the most efficient way for most people to achieve the body they want. An MRT sessions takes 40 to 60 minutes start to finish. It burns calories during and after the session, gives our body a reason to hold onto that precious lean muscle mass, and even build a little in the process too. Traditional methods take more time for less or similar at best results. And honestly, for most people it's plain not fun to spend an hour on an elliptical. My question for you is this: if there's a better way to accomplish your goals faster, why not utilize it?

My Take on Traditional Weight Lifting

As with any sort of really giant topic like this, the answer is that 'it depends'. It depends because each person has different goals, but for the sake of fat loss, I think a minimal portion of time should be spend doing exclusively strength/traditional weight training. At our gym, we host multiple types of sessions, one of them being a FitCamp—Strength type session. While we do slow things down a bit and utilize more muscle and more weight with this type of session, we are still keeping things metabolic by adding in mini circuits, strength circuits, and not taking long breaks between sets. Contrast this to traditional weight training, and it's easy to see how it's a different setup.

If someone is looking to gain as much muscle as possible in a short period of time, or an athlete needs to go up in a weight class by putting on slabs of muscle, traditional weight/strength training methods are going to be utilized. Most of our clients, however, are interested in fat loss, just like you, so having 'strength based' sessions instead of strength only sessions accomplish this goal for all of our members, and it'll do the same for you.

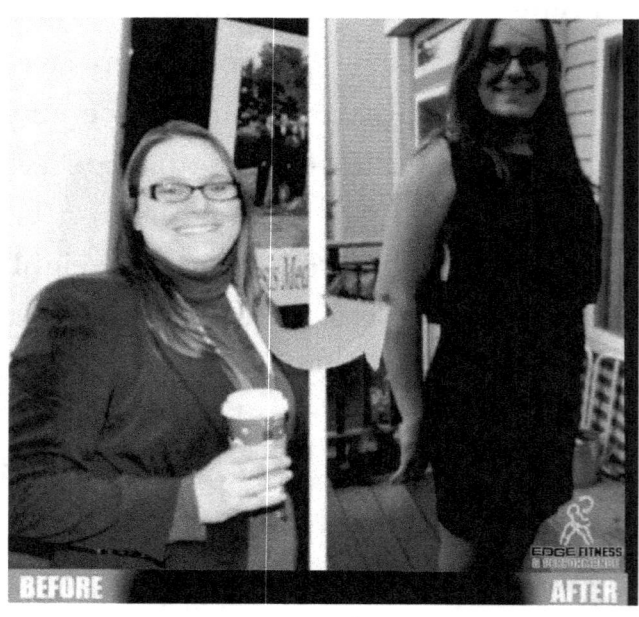

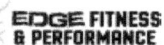

9 Six Fat Loss Training Myths Exposed

What are some myths about losing fat that need to be laid to rest?

Although I could write a sequel to this book with myths, I'd rather keep things simple and to the point. Let's go with six.

1. The first is that **more is better**. The reality about more is better is that it's garbage. 'Better' is the only thing that

can qualify as `better'. What I mean by that is stop doing 'stuff' just for the sake of doing it, and start doing things that are actually going to bring you closer to your goals.

If you start doing a really hard ab workout video that you really feel, take a look at it for four to eight weeks, and take a look at why you're doing it in the first place. Did you lose inches in your waist? Do your abs look better? Does your lower back (a key proponent/reason for ab training!) feel better/stronger/less pain? If the answer is 'yes' to any one or more of these questions, then you should go for it. But if it's not, then why does it matter if you 'feel it'? Or, if you are adding a calorie counting wrist watch to track your calories but you are still drinking a bottle of wine every night, the problem is not the wrist watch or the tracking of the calories. You know what the problem is and that's what you should focus on fixing. The simple answer is that adding these things make us feel better, but if they don't actually make us better, they are just taking up time and energy we could spend elsewhere getting more results.

Some people think that adding more and more things into their daily routine is what's going to make progress faster and that's simply not true. Many times we need to look at what we are already doing and modify or simplify from that. If you're already doing MRT 3-4x/week, being generally active for the rest of the week, and are tracking your calories, what more do you need to add? What more can you? It'd be much easier to give up your mocha-frappe-chino taking up 400 calories every morning then adding in anything else. Simply, minimize, and stop thinking more is going to be better.

2. The second is that **losing weight is what matters**. We touched on this a little bit in our introduction but to elaborate: Too many clients we see are slaves to the scale at first. This alone isn't a huge problem (okay, it is, but lets pretend it's not) but it's what they begin comparing to that makes a big difference. They'll start comparing their current weight to the weight that they were when they were in high school, college, etc. This is a mistake for a series of reasons:

- The first is that most people have what we call `imagination inflation'. This is a sort of historical exaggeration that makes us feel like we used to be more successful then we are right now. This happens all the time with former lifters or football players who come into the gym. They'll say "oh, I used to bench 365 when I weighed 200 pounds," when in reality they were 220 pounds and only benched 300, which is a pretty dramatic difference. Overtime, you tend to exaggerate the story a little bit here and there, you tend to forget and not have good records because you probably weren't tracking and the end result is that you don't really remember correctly. Thinking you weighed 125lbs while working out 3x/week and eating whatever you wanted is very different then weighing 135lbs while working out every day and eating 1000 calories, but this is exactly what our imagination tends to do to us over time. This is why i'll make such a big case against people talking about the weight they used to be back in high school.

- The other thing is that life does happen and it gets in the way, so rather than trying to fight through that (which is going to be impossible for most of us) it is better to just roll with what we have right now. If you were 120 pounds, or at least remember yourself being 120 pounds in high school, that doesn't matter anymore. The only thing that matters is what you weigh now and that you want to lose fat and look and feel better. Besides is it possible that in the last 15 to 20 years that you might have more muscle, you might have more bone density, or you might have just a couple extra pounds that you are not going to get rid of because you are not 17 or 18 anymore, or you might have had a child or two or three. This changes the game big time, and recognizing where you're at right now is critical. The first step towards making long term change and long term results is to recognize those things and to be okay with them.

Losing fat is what matters. Not what you used to weigh. Not what you think you need to weigh now. Not what the scale says. You need to refocus your energy and you efforts into burning fat and being the best YOU that you can be at this moment right now. It may be that you can and WILL indeed get in the best shape you've ever been in. If you follow all the steps in this book, you   will definitely get in the best shape you can get in right now. The point is, if   you are comparing to a former you that might not have ever existed, when will   it ever be enough?

3.   The third myth that needs to be laid to rest is that **100% effort is needed to lose fat**. All the things we've talked about so far in this book are pretty simple and straight forward. There's really nothing revolutionary, there's really maybe   nothing that is completely new to you (although I hope there is because I hate reading books where I learn nothing). If there is something brand spankin' new to you that's great...but if not, what does that tell you? It simply means that we need more implementation of all the information that we probably already know, and less ideas. We have so much information at the tips of our fingers that more information is not

going to do us much good. What we need now is to take action on what we have and if that means that we put out 80% or 90% effort all the time we are still going to get significantly better results than if we were busy trying to figure out how to put 100% in.

The reality is that no one is perfect and you don't need to be in order to really lose fat— you just need to be pretty darn good most of the time.

4. The fourth myth is that **getting very lean is what everybody wants**. This one is honestly what bogs me down the most. Too many people take a look at online advertisements, magazines, cover models and things of that nature and decide that's what they want to look like. Well, the reality is they've never looked like that before and they probably really don't care to look like that. *"Oh if you only knew…"* If you

have 50 pounds to lose and you also want to look like a cover model, then stop thinking about looking like a cover model at first and start thinking about how you are going to lose the first 10 and then the first 20 and so on and so forth to hit that 50lbs of fat lost. If a year or two down the line you decide that you want to get super lean and look like a cover model, then that's the goal at that point. Until then, it's more important to focus on step by step improving yourself. At a certain point you might realize that it's not worth getting leaner. You might be working out more then you like, restricting your calories or food intake lower then you want, or simply neglecting other aspects of your life in order to hit that cover model goal.

To get extremely lean and look like those cover model takes a ton of work.

Once you're fit, once you've accomplished the initial goal, you have to ask yourself how much more you want out of your fitness journey. For many of my clients, losing a few pant sizes, losing some body fat, and feeling better is plenty! Others go 'the distance', and that's great too—just realize it's a different game altogether.

5. The fifth myth is that **excessive protein consumption or lifting (like weight lifting and lifting heavy weights) is going to make you bulky**. The joke out there is that it's cupcakes that make you bulky, not chicken breast or protein shakes. This is kind of a funny comparison, but also technically true. We tend to worry so much about things that we know are good for our bodies and then justify the bad. We know additional protein is going to make us feel fuller, it's going to help save our lean muscle mass; we know

that it's to build muscle and not necessarily to build fat. With lifting, we know it's going to increase our bone density, we know it's going to increase our lean muscle mass, we know it's going to increase our posture, we know it's going to burn calories, so what do we do? We only focus on the novel concept that it *might* make us bulky. Yet when we drink wine and eat cupcakes, have pizza and a bunch of alcoholic beverages we don't think `oh, that's going to make us bulky'. The end result always comes down to this: one is going to have you lean and looking better, the other one is going to have you add extra inches on your waist line.

Protein and weight lifting and lifting heavy, especially for females, are not what make you bulky. It's what helps you get lean, helps you burn body fat and it's what helps preserve the rest of the muscle mass that you have on your body and it might add a little bit. In nearly a decade of helping clients get lean through strength training, I have yet to see anyone get bulky from the programs that we put out. Chances are good you are similar to the clients we've helped, and your body is just waiting to change if you do the right things!

6. The sixth and final myth of fat loss that needs to be exposed is **eating sensibly is overrated**. I guess that depends on your definition of sensible. When I think sensible, I think of things on both sides of the coin. On one hand, eating a bad breakfast (think chocolate chip pancakes and eggs benedict, something really tough to fit into your daily calories or fat, protein, carb breakdown) and then making the rest of the day work by being a little more

strict, and a little more boring is sensible the rest of the day.

The idea that you need to eat sensibly all the time is pretty tough to reconcile with. People go on vacation and think `oh, I can't eat this or I can't eat that' or they are at their son's birthday party and they don't want to have a slice of cake. The problem with this logic is that eventually when you cave, you are going to cave hard. What you need to do in order to have long lasting success is learn how to track your eating. You need to learn how to maintain good habits and how to jump back on when all that stuff goes out the window, because at some point it will. Rather then worry about never failing, worry about what you are going to do when you do fail. It is good to eat sensibly most of the time but for the most part we need to remember that we are all human, we have other lives other than just losing fat and getting lean. In order to accomplish these things we need to make sure that we are keeping everything balanced and in perspective.

Are you interested in training at Edge Fitness?
Call us directly at (773) 577-1190 to get
your free, no obligation, consultation and to see how
we can help you lose fat faster and for good.

Or email me at michael@edgestrength.com
for more information on how
we can help you start getting results now!

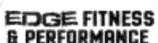
EDGE FITNESS
& PERFORMANCE

---

10 How to Choose the Right Gym for Maximum Results

How I Would Choose a Gym

To figure out how I would choose a gym, I would actually start with three things that I wouldn't use as a base when comparing for gyms. In other words, I'd rule out gyms with three benchmarks of criteria that'll help me narrow down the gym I want to get results at.

The first thing and the thing that I am sure everyone likes to use as the main comparison factor is **price**. Now, before people grab their pitch forks and go up in arms I want to say this: you are not just buying gym membership. The people that think they are just buying a gym membership are setting themselves up failure. You are buying a new life; you are buying years onto your life; you are buying a chance to get lean and a chance to get healthy and not just be a grandmother, but be one that sprints after her grandkids.

It's pretty hard to put a price on that, but to try, just start looking at doctors' bills, the cost for high blood pressure medication or type II diabetes medication, and insurance premiums for being unhealthy. When you start to compare that to a slightly more expensive gym membership it becomes a little bit easier to see. There have been multiple studies and articles that show the 'high cost of low cost gym memberships' that you can view, but the gist of it is that low cost gym businesses not only thrive on, but literally cannot survive without people who pay the membership and do not show up. They need you to fail and to pay them money while you do it.

Paying a higher cost for a gym membership should only matter if you have an accountability factor built in. Is a coach or trainer responsible for checking in on you if you're not showing up? Do they know your story? Do they care? you may not think these things matter, but at Edge Fitness & Performance we have helped dozens of people jump back ON the wagon after falling off simply by caring enough to check in on them. Most people need a support system in place to achieve fat loss, and what better way then having one built into their membership?

The second thing I wouldn't use is **session size** of each session to determine if the gym is right for me, and the reason for this is simple. I used to think one-on-one training was always the best way to train a client and get results, period. Then we started to do group personal training at our facility, *Edge Fitness and Performance,* and the thing that we immediately noticed is that people were coming to us from their one-on-one trainers and still felt like they were getting better attention and a better education on how to lose fat. What's more important is who is coaching you. Are they helping correct your form? Do they care if you miss a session? Are they excited for you to get better? These matter more then if you're sweating next to another person or not.

What I would focus on instead of session size is a client to coach ratio. At our gym we like to have a 10:1 client to coach ratio most of the time with a few coaches being able to go up to 15:1. Any more than that and the coaching quality is tough to achieve. There are plenty of big bootcamps to choose from that are low cost, high membership count. I can't and won't speak for other gyms, but at Edge Fitness, you are much more then a number and a dollar sign.

The last thing I wouldn't use when it comes to choosing a gym that's right for me would be **the amenities**. The reality is that most people don't use amenities and that's what they are paying a premium on bigger box gym membership for. It's great to have a pool, it's great to have a basketball court, and it's great to have a hot tub. But it's time to do a self audit— when was the last time you actually used any of those things? When is the next time you are going to? Did playing basketball ever help you get results in fat loss? How about the hot tub? If you're holding onto the membership with the hopes that you one day hang out in the hot tub for 20 minutes, you need to find a gym that is actually going to help you get results and guide you in the right direction on your path to getting lean.

How You'll Know When You're in the Right Gym

The first thing you should feel is like **you are welcomed**. If people are giving you the cold shoulder, if personal trainers or coaches seem like they are disinterested in helping you, you are probably in the wrong place so turn and run, and run fast. The good news is sprinting away from the negativity might be the best thing they do to help you get results!

The second thing that I would focus on is: **are you being treated like just another number or are you being treated like a person?** You can learn how to become a better coach, but you can't easily learn to be a better person who genuinely cares more. Our hiring process is lengthy (we onboard our coaches for months to make sure they are a good fit for our clients and our culture) because we need to make sure all of our coaches/trainers actually care about each and every one of our members. At Edge Fitness, we make it a priority to not only greet everyone by name, but actually know about their life, about their kids, the good and the bad happenings, the things that they did over the weekend and by doing this we ensure that people feel like a family; which leads me to the next thing I'd look for when choosing a gym.

It is important to **have a family atmosphere in the gym**. Warehouse or more industrial style gyms are definitely gaining popularity right now, and they do offer some advantages over typical health club settings, but they shouldn't turn people away. They shouldn't make people feel like they are not welcome because they are not at a certain fitness level yet.

Everyone should be welcome in a good gym. Even if I was coming in at a higher level then others, I would choose a gym that was welcoming to everyone. A good coach should be able to help me, and a brand new client, both get results.

The last thing I would focus on is **the actual coaching and the knowledge the coaching staff presents**. Sometimes high energy sessions are great, but were you actually coached? Did someone actually cue and give you tips to take away and have better form; or were they just cheering you on? I've been to other gyms where the energy was high, the workouts were really cool, but I wasn't helped once with anything. I know some of our current clients have been in that boat as well. When I am hiring a coach or paying a gym membership that includes coaching and personal training or group training, I would focus on what they are doing to help make me better. Are they giving me actual knowledge or are they just being a cheerleader? If I wanted a cheerleader, I could have a family member cheer me on in my basement gym; if I want someone to coach me, I'm going to find a gym that can do it. Keep this in mind when you go to a high energy place that's doing cross training—remember, doing more for the sake of doing it doesn't get results. Make sure you choose a gym that has a coaching staff that will do things to make you better, not just sweaty and sore. Remember, more is not better – better is better. Is the gym that you are choosing helping you get better or is it just having you doing more stuff?

Bootcamp Training vs Personal Training

It really depends on the person seeking out help, and on what level of bootcamp trainer or personal trainer you are choosing. Like I mentioned before, we've had many people come from one-on-

one trainers, who felt like they were wasting their money. They come to us, a small group training facility, and experience much better results, much better coaching and much better atmosphere, and they also do all of this at a lower cost. So, if you are going to pay for one-on-one training every single minute should be focused 100% on you. There are certainly one on one trainers who do a great job at this.

To be honest, even if you are in group training atmosphere, 100% of the effort and the focus should be on each and every client the entire time. If it's not, you need to ask yourself what are you paying for: to watch your personal trainer, bootcamp instructor or coach text on the phone and flirt with the girl on the machine next to you? Or are you paying for someone to help you get better and lose fat faster?

Those are the things that I would look at when choosing a gym. At *Edge Fitness and Performance* we pride ourselves on providing all of these things for our members. Our goal is to be the best part of our member's day, every day by caring more, and by providing better results in a welcoming atmosphere.